Chakra Breathing

Pathway to Energy, Harmony and
Self-Healing

Helmut G. Sieczka

Chakra Breathing

Pathway to Energy, Harmony and Self-Healing

LifeRhythm

Translated from the German and edited
by Jalaja Bonheim Ph.D.
Photographs: Fotostudio Wagner, Germany

Library of Congress Cataloging-in-Publication Data
Sieczka, Helmut G.
    [Chakra. English]
    Chakra Breathing; breath as pathway to energy, harmony and self-healing/Helmut G. Sieczka: [translated from the German and edited by Jalaja Bonheim...].
ISBN 0-94-0795-11-6
1. Chakras. 2. Yoga. 3. Exercise—Miscellanea. 4. Healing—Miscellanea.
I. Title.
BF 1990.S51513 1993   94-3642
613.7'046--dc20

Copyright © LifeRhythm 1994
PO Box 806
Mendocino CA 95460 USA
Telephone (707) 937-1825 Fax (707) 937-3052

Printed in the United States of America

Table of Contents

Whoever nourishes himself with air becomes radiant like a god and lives a long life.

Confucius

Two blessings doth our breath bestow: drawing in air, then letting it go; first we are pressured, then delivered; the strands of life are thus wondrously mingled.

The Singer's Book, Talisman
Goethe

Introduction

We were driven out of paradise, and out of the consciousness of oneness, not by accident, but rather because of our soul's conscious choice—a choice crucial to our spiritual evolution.

We left, or perhaps, fell from the knowledge of oneness, so that by following the path of learning and self-discovery, we might eventually return to the source as more mature, spiritually evolved beings. Therefore, our experience within the world of duality and individuation should be viewed as a process of growth, purification, and realization. The purpose of life is to set out on the path, and, following that path finally return to the original state of union with more inner wealth and awareness to contribute to life as a whole.

Yorgason's simple, clear words in *The Monument* outline the essential meaning of a human being's incarnation:

Before sending his children down to earth, God handed each one a bundle of carefully selected problems. These problems, he promised everyone with a smile, are yours alone. No-one else will experience the blessing these problems will bestow upon you. And you alone possess the special gifts and talents which can transform these problems into your devoted servants. Now, dive into your birth and into forgetfulness. Know that my love for you is limitless. These problems I give you in token of my love. With their help, you will create your life as a monument symbolizing the love you bear me, your Father.

Actually, problems do not exist; only situations which we are not yet capable of comprehending and accepting because our consciousness is not yet sufficiently developed. For this reason, we tend to deny, ignore and repress problems so tenaciously. Until we face them, we have no choice but to constantly sacrifice our energy to them, serving them like slaves. For in our lives, nothing can continue to exist unless we feed it with our attention and mental affirmation.

Today, you may find yourself able to emotionally

accept situations which, only a few years ago, seemed torturous—acceptance being the ability to witness something without judging it. By grappling with the situation, you have learned to deal with it, and as a result, your mind can accept it. This is what problem-solving is all about. Do not expect your environment to do this for you. Rather, your own personal growth process will enable you to solve the problem on the inner level. Thus, problem solving involves an expansion of consciousness.

Many mystics and spiritual teachers claim that we exist eternally, and that we never cease to evolve; that the human being is a thought form of God made manifest and endowed with freedom of choice. How we choose to live our life and what we choose to express through it is up to each one of us. To live is to receive the gift of being. Though life challenges us to raise our consciousness, unfortunately we have, to a large degree, lost touch with the truly essential aspects of life.

In these times of career-induced stress and hyper-competitiveness, it is difficult to find quiet and medi-tative moments. The craving for power and prestige has increased, as well. Though, truly speaking, we never have and never will own anything permanently, many people devote all their energy to the pursuit of success and possessions. We are, at most, transient guests—renters perhaps, certainly not the landlords. We wait until it is too late. Only when we have exhausted ourselves and realize that something inside is broken and no longer works are we ready to turn inward, returning to ourselves. Unfortunately, the body's messages and its cries for help are often ignored or numbed with medication, allowing us to keep moving in a wrong direction until irreparable damage has occurred.

We should start turning inward, allowing the natural balance of energies to be restored. The more centered a life we live, the more often we will be able to experience peace, serenity, and harmony.

The practice of breathing into the chakras can support our journey toward realization and liberation, especially insofar as the emotional and energetic dimensions of our being are concerned. We must keep in mind that permanent joy depends on transcending the dualities of life and rediscovering the oneness of existence. Then, our yearning for joy and wholeness may be fulfilled.

Chapter 1

Energy Blockage Caused by Past Experience

The birth experience

Obviously, outer circumstances must be considered in relation to energy blockages. At birth, we delve into the gross material realm. Scientists and medical researchers have found that an embryo in the mother's womb is already impressionable. Birth is such a core experience because of the concentration of events which, within a very brief span of time, radically transform the baby's reality.

The environment changes: instead of the pleasurable warmth of the embryonic fluid, the child senses the cold. Previously surrounded by the protection of the mother's body, it may now feel incredibly insecure. Therefore, many people try to recreate the sense of oneness experienced within the mother's body by staying in bed or taking long hot baths.

While the embryo receives oxygen through the umbilical cord, a baby must breathe on its own. Often, the umbilical cord is severed too early, preventing the lungs from unfolding gently and gradually. At this point, one may acquire beliefs such as "Breathing is hard work," or "Life is a struggle." The first social interactions, which generally involve the doctor and the midwife, are equally crucial. If the baby is not handled gently, conclusions may be drawn such as "Other people will hurt me," or "People cannot be trusted." When babies are separated from the mother too soon, before they have had time to adjust to the new environment, later symptoms may include a sense of insecurity and alienation, a lack of primal self-confidence and separation anxiety.

I shall discuss these symptoms further in the context of the various chakras. If you are interested in further study of this subject, I recommend *Birth without Violence*, by Frederick Leboyer, and *Rebirthing* by Phil Laut and Jim Leonard.

Childhood

Sociologists and psychologists have repeatedly emphasized the importance of a child's first years. Nonetheless, many children grow up in an environment in which adults fail to explain their behavior and their reactions. We all gather many painful and unresolved memories of times when we had to deal with negative belief systems, inappropriate reactions of those around us, threats, rejection, loss or lack of love, attention and tenderness. Such experiences leave obvious scars on body, soul, and spirit.

These early events, as well the suffering caused by our fear of not surviving, may surface in adulthood as unspecific anxieties, self-defeating habits, physical tension, emotional disturbance, depression and serious health problems.

The most important psychic wounds to consider in this context are fear of not surviving and fear of loss. Repressed emotions and unresolved pain decrease one's level of awareness, physical health, vitality and life energy. We can easily understand how suffering, whether physical, mental or emotional, influences the entire energy system of the human being and prevents the free flow of life energies.

Healing the wounds and taking responsibility

If, with the help of conscious breathing, we manage to integrate and thus dissolve all the fears and the pain which we carry around—the unfinished business of our inner life—then we will be able to remember our true origins and simultaneously experience a sense of oneness with the entire universe.

At this point, I would like to point out that we ourselves have chosen both the time and place of our incarnation and our parents. There is no point in faulting someone else. Evolution, in the sense of becoming a whole human being, is not possible until we become response-able, that is, able to respond to the events of our life without blaming others for our destiny.

As mentioned previously, conflict, fear, and pain must be healed before liberation can occur. Unfortunately, we tend to ignore our own easily accessible self-healing abilities. By increasing our intake of oxygen, we can strengthen the inner life-force and absorb increasingly subtle and pure forms of energy. These, in turn, allow us to view the problem from a different and often higher vantage point, and to dissolve its negative implications. The resolution of an inner conflict always frees both our energy and our breathing. Our personal vibration (the microcosm) becomes aligned and harmoniously integrated with the primal vibration of the macrocosm. The duller and denser a body, or, in other words, the slower its basic rate of vibration—the greater a person's distance from the realm of oneness and the light source of their being. This is the significance of the word *religion*, which means returning to the source and communing with being itself

We all naturally yearn for cosmic oneness, for the feeling of security and fulfillment. Consciously or unconsciously, we seek to establish connection with the whole. Through the course of a life-time, this longing moves us through many phases. By surrendering to the soul's urging, we experience ever deepening levels of insight.

It is possible to rediscover the joy and ecstasy of life, and the odds may be better than we believe.

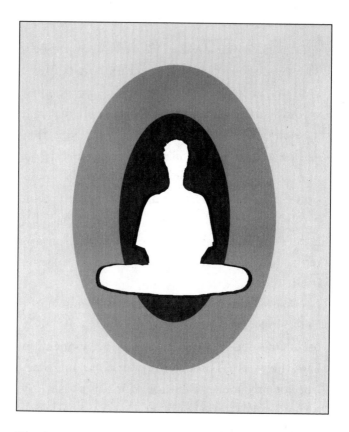

The human aura consists of four layers, listed from the innermost to the outermost:

- ⬛ The etheric body
- ⬛ The astral body
- ⬛ The mental body
- ⬜ The causal body

Chapter 2

The Subtle Bodies

A few comments on the purpose and functions of the subtle energy system are necessary before we proceed to the actual breathing practices.

The most important building blocks of the human energy system are:

1. The subtle bodies
2. The energy centers or chakras;
3. The energetic connections or channels.

Apart from the tangible and visible physical body, we possess four other subtle, invisible energy bodies:

1. The etheric body
2. The astral body
3. The mental body
4. The causal body

Like the chakras, each energy body also possesses its own unique vibratory frequency. The energy bodies interpenetrate one another and are in lively communication with each other.

The etheric body

The etheric body resembles the physical body most closely in terms of its vibratory frequency and size. It envelops the visible body with a four to six inch thick cloud of energy, creating a protective barrier against bacteria and toxins. The etheric body plays an important part in defining an individual's level of vitality and outward appearance.

It is nourished and energized via the root chakra (the earth) and the solar plexus (the sun). These are the two sources from which the etheric body receives energy, stores it and channels a constant stream of energy to the physical body. Stress, negative thinking, unhealthy diet, and the misuse of alcohol and nicotine all deplete the etheric body. By regularly spending time outdoors and in nature, you can charge the etheric body and strengthen its protective shield.

The astral body

The astral body vibrates at a somewhat higher frequency than the etheric body. It is responsible for the emotional realm and for certain aspects of our personality. Depending on our developmental level, the radiant aura of the astral body may extend out one, or even several yards, from the physical body.

The astral body is the medium of all feelings and emotions. This body mirrors our fear, aggression, joy and love with the utmost clarity and facilitates our emotional communication with others. Our feelings and emotions are most readily perceived around the area of the solar plexus, which also provides the astral body with nourishment.

By way of the astral level we establish a connection (often unconscious) with deeper levels of our own psyche. This is the source of interpersonal attraction and aversion.

The mental body

The mind or mental body is limited in its capacity to clear unresolved emotional issues. Ultimately, this can occur only via the causal body, or with the help of integrative processes.

The mental body is the site of ideas and thoughts. Its vibratory frequency is higher as well as lighter and more radiant than that of the etheric and the astral bodies. The mental body bears responsibility for our creative thought processes, for how we respond to information transmitted by the astral and the causal bodies, and how we utilize this information for our spiritual evolution.

We can actively feed energy into the mental body by choosing a lifestyle that supports the unfolding of our consciousness and includes meditation, self-acceptance, and grappling with our shadow sides. The mental body is closely related to the third eye and crown chakras. When these two centers are open and balanced, one is able to receive information and messages beyond the scope of the five senses.

The causal body

Among the subtle bodies, the causal body vibrates at the fastest rate. It provides us with an unbroken line of communication with the inner divine, the realm of eternity and pure being. The energetic sources of the causal body, which is also called the spiritual body, lie in the highest vibrational realms of pure love, light, and being. At the level of the causal body, the permanent transformation of all unresolved issues can occur.

Prana

Energy or *prana* is distributed throughout the entire energy system and the energy bodies through the subtle energy channels or *nadis*. Prana is life force and vital or cosmic energy. All that lives contains prana. Prana is stored within air, food, water and sunlight. Prana enlivens matter. Prana is the fuel that heightens the vibratory frequency of the chakras and of the energy bodies. Prana is primal energy, and should not be confused with oxygen.

Prana flows throughout the entire energy system. The nadis form the basis for a vital exchange of energy between the chakras and the etheric, astral, mental and causal bodies. Ancient Tibetan scriptures claim that there are up to 72,000 energy channels in the human body.

Chapter 3

The Seven Chakras

The chakras

Chakras are centers of energy and consciousness within the subtle etheric body. They are the human being's main focal points of vital energy. Chakra is a Sanskrit word meaning 'whirl' or 'wheel.' Chakras constantly spin in a circular motion.

The spinal column supports the complex interconnections between the chakras. Their harmonious co-operation provides the foundation for physical and psychic health as well as the human being's mental and spiritual evolution.

In the average human adult, the chakras look like small, three-dimensional circles, two to four inches in diameter, on the surface of the etheric body. Except for the seventh chakra, they all correspond to nerve bundles located in the physical body throughout the spine. Without these energy centers, the physical body could not exist.

Chakras are cone-shaped openings, receivers, transmitters and centers of power, which receive vital or cosmic energy and distribute it to the subtle bodies and the physical organs.

Each center possesses its own unique quality of energy and vibrational frequency that reflects the quality of our thoughts and feelings. A chakra's vibration also indicates the level of our spiritual evolution and determines the quality of energy received and transformed.

We know that each chakra relates directly to the body parts surrounding it, and also has an effect on behavior and mental development.. So far, only visionaries and psychics are able to perceive the chakras. However, anyone can activate and balance them with the help of simple yet extremely effective breathing techniques. As a result of practicing them, you will experience an increase in your awareness and sensitivity.

When we nourish the chakras regularly and consciously with the energy of our breath, they begin to radiate a brilliant, pulsating light. At the same time, the surrounding organs and cells receive a greater quantity of energy and are brought into balance.

A general analysis of the seven chakras shows that the first two chakras are responsible for physical energies. The three middle chakras deal with the development of an individual's personality and personal strength, while the third eye and crown chakras determine one's mental attitudes and evolution, clarity of thought and awareness of the principle of universal love.

The root chakra is located opposite the crown chakra, and opens toward the earth. The spleen chakra, the solar plexus, heart, throat and third eye centers open toward the front, while the crown chakra opens upward, according to its function.

The seven chakras play an important part at each stage of human development. As a person evolves, each respective chakra opens and unfolds further.

Preventing disease by raising the vibrational frequency

The higher one's vibrational frequency, the easier it is to prevent physical and mental disturbances. Fear, negative thoughts and powers cannot take hold when one is flooded with pure energy and light.

The prana energy released through the practice of conscious breathing will greatly improve our mental and physical health. When our energy flows without obstruction, we perceive situations differently and can ascend to a more evolved level of human existence.

Honest self-appraisal

Naturally, any book is limited in its ability to respond to the reader's potential questions, especially when the subject is as complex as the human energy system. The following descriptions and interpretations may not always apply to your own case. However, they can help you develop a new way of perceiving disease by relating to it from a different, energetic perspective.

As you reflect on your own state of body and mind, you may be taken aback by the accuracy of some of the following descriptions. Though self-discovery is not always pleasurable, our shadow aspects need to be integrated, as well. I would advise anyone who is experiencing an overwhelmingly intensive process of transformation to consider all available therapeutic possibilities. Both body-oriented and verbal forms of therapy are valuable and may complement each other.

Chakra sounds

Each chakra radiates a specific vibration, comparable to the vibrations of musical instruments. The first or root chakra vibrates slowly, emitting a deep note. The higher the chakra is located in the body, the faster and subtler are its vibrations. Therefore each chakra can also resonate with sounds and vibrations outside of the body.

We have utilized the knowledge of these frequencies by creating a chakra breathing tape, which includes a sound for each chakra. (See page 93 for ordering information.)

Chapter 4

Symptoms of Reduced or Open Energy Flow in the Chakras

First chakra

Root chakra

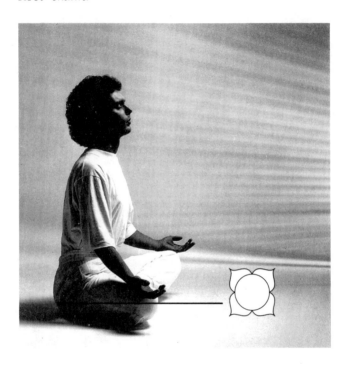

Location: Perineum/Coccyx
Element: Earth
Color: Dark red
Corresponding glands: Adrenal glands

Reduced energy flow
Mental symptoms:

Lack of self-assertiveness and confidence in life, difficulty in finding a sense of direction, frequent feelings of insecurity, inexplicable vague feelings of anxiety, constant worry, shaky connection to reality and to the earth, existential fears around survival, mental rigidity.

Physical symptoms:

Generally weak constitution, complaints in the leg area, for instance veinal problems; postural problems relating to the spine, problems with teeth, gums, bones and joints, inhibited rejuvenation of blood and cells, frequent injuries.

Open energy flow

Alertness and clarity in daily life, strong motivation and perseverance, firm rootedness in life, strong physical and mental resilience, high level of physical confidence and self-assurance, firm connection with the earth and with nature, love of life, contentment and inner peace.

Second chakra
Navel chakra

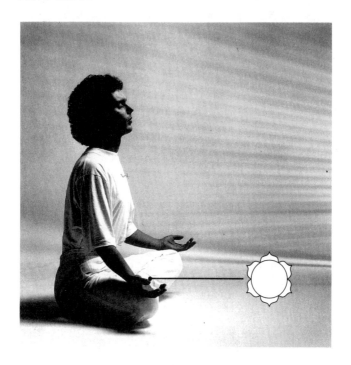

Location: Sacral vertebra, about two inches below
the navel
Element: Water
Color: Orange
Corresponding gland: Gonads

Reduced energy flow

Mental symptoms:

Plagued by doubt, lack of interest, indecisiveness and lethargy in daily life, depression, low energy, clinging to the past, materialism, physical and sexual inhibitions.

Physical symptoms:

Shallow and irregular breathing, frequent low energy, irritability and chronic disturbances of the central nervous system, nervousness, diseases of the gallbladder and liver, lower back complaints, constipation, migraines, problems with sexual potency.

Open energy flow

Vitality and sexual energy, a harmonious sex life, a well-balanced physical constitution, deep feelings of connection and security toward oneself and others, rich emotional life and developed sense of empathy, zest for action, love of touch and caresses; calmness, strong nerves and a cheerful outlook, well-balanced gallbladder and liver, constant body temperature.

Third chakra

Solar plexus

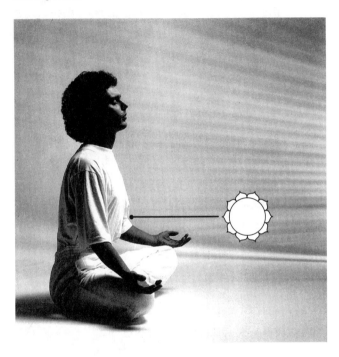

Location: Solar plexus, third lumbar vertebra
Colors: Yellow and gold
Corresponding gland: Pancreas

Reduced energy flow

Mental symptoms:

Defensiveness, insecurity, frequent feelings of boredom, repressed emotions, inexplicable sadness, listlessness and apathy, inability to surrender, yearning for a conflict-free environment, extreme hunger for power, egotism, unrefined emotionality.

Physical symptoms:

Stiffness, rigidity, and muscular tensions, stomach and digestive problems, problems in the lower back.

Open energy flow

A sense of well-being, motivated action, determination, trust in change, centeredness, willingness to overcome physical and mental limitation, ability to resolve conflicts, in touch with one's emotions, contentment and trust, self-acceptance, a sense of lightness, clarity and fulfillment, strong digestive system.

Fourth chakra

Heart chakra

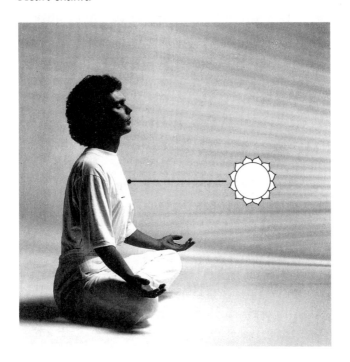

Location: Fifth thoracic vertebra
Element: Air
Color: Light red
Corresponding gland: Thymus

Reduced energy flow

Mental symptoms:

Loss of awareness of one's deepest and truest feelings, closed heart, difficulties in relating and lack of contact, difficulties in receiving love and affection, lack of connection to one's normal life rhythms, extreme disharmony between thinking and feeling, overwhelming negative thoughts, distaste for life.

Physical symptoms:

Collapsed shoulders, flat chest (commonly a sense of an iron girdle around one's chest), general breathing problems, diseases of the lungs and the skin, nervous heart ailments.

Open energy flow

Confidence in relationships, developed sensitivity; high level of empathy, openness, trust and love for oneself and others, generosity and helpfulness, a high degree of flexibility and adaptability, physical balance and health, natural and lively vital rhythms, compassion (as opposed to pity), optimism, cheerfulness and warmth, inner tranquility, harmony, healthy blood and a well functioning circulatory system.

Fifth chakra
Throat chakra

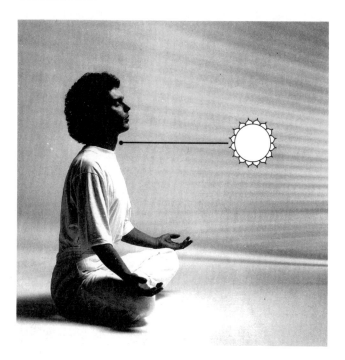

Location: First cervical vertebra
Element: Ether
Color: Light blue
Corresponding gland: Thyroid

Reduced energy flow

Mental symptoms:

Speech and communication problems such as stuttering, difficulties with vocalization, inhibited creative expressiveness, insecurity concerning one's creative powers, desire to abnegate responsibility and maintain the role of a child, powerful yearning for safety and stability, feeling overwhelmed, stubbornness, reclusive life-style, self-hatred and distaste for life.

Physical symptoms:

Exhaustion, digestive and weight problems, frequent colds, sores throats and throat infections, tension in the shoulders, neck, and back of the head, possible stiffness and rigidity of the arms and hands.

Open energy flow

High degree of responsibility, creativity, wealth of ideas, good communication skills and expressiveness, joy in giving, a sense of abundance, freedom and independence, moving with the flow of life, highly developed personality structure, the sense of being accepted, a strong immune system.

Sixth chakra
Third eye chakra

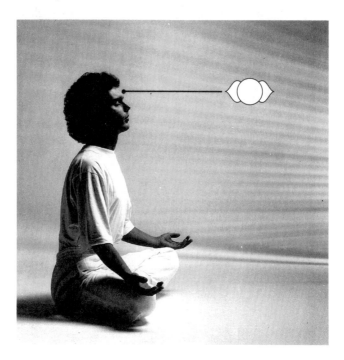

Location: Center of forehead
Element: Light
Colors: Violet and purple
Corresponding gland: Pituitary

Reduced energy flow
Mental symptoms:

Problems with concentration and self-identity, fear of criticism and judgement, strongly controlling behavior, denial of reality, repetitive thoughts and inner dialogues, forgetfulness, unrelenting pressure to achieve, low level of trust in one's emotions and perceptions.

Physical symptoms:

Imbalance of all paired bodily parts and organs, headaches, eye and vision problems, near and far-sightedness.

Open energy flow

Balance of all paired bodily parts and organs, a sense of centeredness, acceptance of the pairs of opposites, balance of feminine and masculine qualities, a strong connection with one's soul, self-knowledge, the gift of intuitive vision, contact with one's inner guidance, openness to spiritual experience, strong powers of the mind and will.

Seventh chakra

Crown chakra

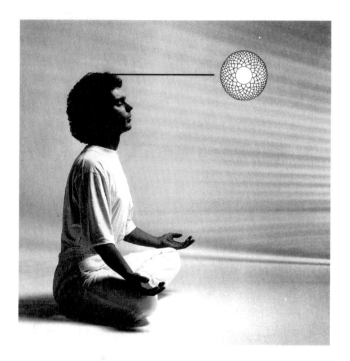

Location: Crown
Colors: White, violet and gold
Corresponding gland : Pineal

Reduced energy flow

Mental symptoms:

Undeveloped sense of wholeness and basic trust, overly strong ego-boundaries, excessive trust in rationality and analysis, constant activity, lack of confidence in one's intuitive powers, intellectual defenses against universal energies and powers.

Physical symptoms:

Ailments of the genital organs, adrenal glands, thyroid and parathyroid glands; general ailments of the muscular system.

Open energy flow

Experiences of cosmic oneness, a sense of connection with both the visible and the invisible planes, pure consciousness, extreme clarity, strong feelings of wholeness and oneness, potential for profound healing and restructuring of body and mind, experiences that transcend time and space, contact with one's spirit, experiences of *satori* and enlightenment.

Chapter 5

Introduction to Chakra Breathing Practices

The breath

Breathing is a continuously flowing, rhythmic motion. Everything changes constantly, but our breath remains a faithful companion throughout life's journey.

Breath is the most important bridge between body and spirit. Ancient Sanskrit uses the world *Atman*, which means something akin to both spirit and breath. The Latin word for spirit is *spiritus*, while the word for breathing is *spirare*. Another related word is 'inspiration,' which literally means inhalation. In Greek, *psyche* means both breath and spirit. Eastern Indians speak of *prana*, the universal life force.

Our own language contains additional idioms that underscore the significance of breathing. We speak of "holding our breath" in anticipation, of a sight "taking our breath away," or of "gasping with horror."

Peaceful breath—peaceful mind

As we all know, a nervous person breathes differently than a calm one. Most people breathe too shallowly and irregularly; their breathing pattern is disturbed. Generally, children are still able to breathe naturally and correctly. Their breath flows easily and fully, following its natural rhythm.

Our "normal" breathing—its speed, rhythm and depth—reveals our current mental and physical state. Breathing also reflects our basic relationship to life. Again and again, people are amazed at the accuracy of my description of their basic attitudes, which is based upon a diagnosis of their breathing patterns. Your breath tells the truth. Breathing is linked to the vegetative nervous system. Like a seismograph, it reacts with great sensitivity to every one of life's changes, creating specific breathing patterns. Thus, breathing patterns reflect life's patterns. Today, more people are becoming aware of the interdependence of body, mind, spirit, and breath.

People who breath shallowly and superficially chronically deprive their blood of oxygen. Such a lack of oxygen causes a slight yet pervasive sense of insecurity, and may even result in feelings of being unable to face the demands of living. Deep breathing increases the blood's oxygen level and counteracts anxiety. A complex biofeedback system informs the brain when the entire organism is saturated with oxygen, dissipating fear of not surviving. We now know that 3 times 7 deep breaths suffice to supply up to eight million body cells with oxygen.

Conscious breathing supports clear thinking and a clear mind. Breathing deeply and thoroughly refreshes us and can give us welcome relief in times of stress, perhaps even unlocking the gate to new insight.

The use of breath as a healing tool in ancient cultures

Among many ancient peoples, such as the Incas, Tibetans, Egyptians and Greeks, breathing exercises were taught. The priests, yogis and spiritual healers were aware of the power of breath and used it for the purpose of healing and to raise consciousness.

The diaphragm—seat of the soul

The ancient Greeks believed the diaphragm to be the seat of the soul. The diaphragm is located in the center of the body and connects the upper with the lower body. The two lungs connect the left (feminine/yin) and the right (masculine/yang) halves of the body.

Guidance from the masters

Many religious teachers and mystics were concerned with the meaning of breath. They believed that the experience of breathing leads to the experience of one's true self and the universe.

In the Dead Sea Scrolls—discovered only a few decades ago—Jesus discusses the sacredness of breathing. He says: "We revere the holy breath which is beyond all creation. For behold, the eternal, highest realm of light, where the infinite stars reign, is the realm of air, which we inhale and exhale. And in the moments between inhalation and exhalation, all the mysteries of the eternal garden are hidden. Angel of the air, holy messenger of the earth mother, dive deeply into me, like a swallow dives from the sky, so that I may know the secret of the wind and the music of the stars."

The East Indian meditation teacher Maharishi says: "Through control of our breath we achieve control over the mind, and by controlling the mind we return to the original state of Eden."

The Buddha used conscious breathing in order to achieve enlightenment, the highest state of consciousness. To this very day, Native American Indians as well as the Sufis include breathing practices in their initiation rituals.

Conscious breathing and holistic therapy

It is not surprising to find that long forgotten breathing practices and exercises are now beginning to resurface. Western men and women are rediscovering breath's rejuvenating and healing power. Especially in the context of holistic health, medication, if needed, is often being supplemented by a recommendation to practice conscious breathing.

Facing unfamiliar thoughts, feelings and sensations

A person who has never before directed their focus inward and paid close attention to body and breath, may by startled at how many thoughts crop up.

Endless trains of thought dance around within our mind, as we slowly begin to detach from external impressions and focus inward. We must wait patiently for tranquility and silence to arrive. The more we try to suppress physical sensations, memories and outer images, the more they will insist on being noticed.

The heightening of one's energy level may cause early childhood memories that were long ago locked away in the psyche's unconscious to resurface and manifest through physical and emotional symptoms. After only a few minutes of practice quite harmless symptoms may appear. These may include a light sensation of tingling on the hands, feet, lips, or wherever the body is not completely healthy and balanced. Organs which are frequently undernourished with oxygen may react with sensations of warmth or pressure. You need not be concerned about such reactions. Should you feel dizzy, slow down the speed of your breathing, which will reduce the volume of inhaled air. After continuing for a few more minutes you will find these unfamiliar sensations dissipating.

The process of chakra breathing may cause obvious physical changes. Allow the energy to flow freely, even if unfamiliar sensations should arise. It is advisable to let these reactions unfold fully, without restricting them. Your breathing will lead you exactly where you need to go, and will cause whatever emerges to do so at just the right moment. Have faith in this inner flow of healing power.

In this context, physical tensions and the subtle, generally ignored symptoms of disease should be approached as carriers of information, by which the symptom is trying to attract our attention and awaken our awareness. Please do not ignore such signals, but rather listen to them. They express some hitherto denied or unlived aspect of your being and signify a need for further growth and development.

Developing patience and mindfulness

The Japanese abbot and meditation teacher Shindai Sekigushi taught: "You will find that much time will pass before you are able to take ten breaths without thinking of anything. It took me about three years. When you practice, all kinds of thoughts arise. Memories both pleasant and unpleasant appear, including those which one would prefer never to tell another person, whether in person or in writing. Embarrassing images may pass through one's mind."

Finally Sekigushi concludes: "It is, however, possible to restrain the stream of thoughts which overwhelm the meditating mind, but only if one does not fight them too hard."

Those high achievers who approach breathing and relaxation exercises with expectations of attaining rapid results will never reach their goal. The opening of the inner eye is best supported by an attitude of patience and mindfulness of each moment. Only in a relaxed and calm state can we recognize and know what is truly important.

By consciously following our breath, we allow it to become our teacher. Breath teaches us the laws of giving and taking, the two opposites. Further, it directs our attention towards potential physical-mental and energetic blockages. If we are willing to pay attention to our breathing and be led by it, we gain the gift of increased self-knowledge.

At every point, try to maintain the attitude of observing without judgement. Generally, chakra breathing guides you into the present moment, into joy, peace, and meditation. If you feel any anxiety around doing these exercises, simply allow yourself more time to get accustomed to the heightened energy level. The best option is to find a guide—a breath teacher who is familiar with chakra breathing.

Working with the chakras, we increase our sensitivity and become receptive to new energies. But this opening also leaves us more vulnerable. We may feel concerned about things which others don't even notice. It is essential to relate in a responsible and conscious manner to the higher energies, so as not to harm ourselves by taking on negative vibrations while we are open, or harming others by passing on impure energy to them.

Self-observation and self-correction

On our path toward the truth we encounter many pitfalls, such as the temptation to misuse power, to manipulate others or mislead them for the sake of our own profit. We must constantly question our actions as we move towards union with our spiritual core and source. We must also relearn to trust our own impressions and insights.

Remember: if you are breathing correctly, you will feel a sense of well-being and find the exercises easy to do. Therefore you should constantly monitor how you are breathing and correct yourself if necessary. Basically, there is no right way or wrong way. Like a thermometer, your breath simply indicates your energy level and the degree of consciousness with which you are breathing.

Chapter 6

Practical Guidelines

Basic rules for breathing practice

- Take your time. Experiment until you have found the optimal sitting posture.

- Avoid trying to open the chakras too quickly or forcefully. Activating and harmonizing the chakras requires an attitude of gentle sensing, loosening, and letting go. Ideally, your mental and spiritual evolution should run parallel with the opening of the chakras. Your breathing and your visualizations help initiate the process of activating the chakras, which will open when the time is right.

- Remember the importance of love. Opening the higher chakras without the lower ones is not advisable. We should keep in mind that the heart chakra, the seat of love, is the soul's gateway. If we recognize that our first priority is to grow in love, we will avoid misusing the third eye chakra as an instrument of power over the mind and will.

Rather, we seek the power of the heart. All chakras must be harmonized simultaneously, so that we maintain awareness of any unresolved issues. A permanent connection to the soul develops only after our inner space has been completely purified and a firm relationship to the powers of the heart has been established. Only then can we live from the source.

• Before you start, settle into a meditative state. Notice your present state of mind, and whatever it is, accept it. If you find yourself restless and tense, say to yourself: "Right now, I am restless and tense." Don't judge yourself but rather, accept whatever is. This basic attitude will allow you to gradually move into a meditative state.

• Breathe gently, carefully, evenly and consciously. Don't try to force anything to happen, and be patient with yourself.

• Don't practice breathing exercises immediately after a meal. Allow at least one hour to pass between eating and practicing.

- Find a familiar, undisturbed practice space.
- Make sure you have plenty of time to practice.
- Practice at regular hours; this will help you to integrate the exercises into your daily routines.
- Wear comfortable, loose clothing.
- Take off your jewelry and any metal objects.
- The room you practice in should be well ventilated.
- Don't overtax yourself. Should you become dizzy, stop practicing. Lie down on your back, breath normally, and relax.
- Breathe through your nose. This helps filter the air and purify it of dust, warm it (especially important in cold climates) and moisturize the mucous membranes.
- Whenever you practice, be sure to visualize the chakras closing after having opened them through your breathing.
- If you suffer from heart or circulatory problems, please consult your physician to make sure the suggested exercises are suitable for you.
- If you practice regularly, it will take roughly three to five minutes to activate and purify each

chakra. Your intuition will let you know whether a chakra has been sufficiently charged or not.

Visualization

Visualization is the ability to create an image or a picture in one's imagination. With the help of inner acceptance and affirmation, our mental pictures and ideas can become reality. As the ancient Greek philosopher Aristotle said, "By mind I refer to the power of the soul that thinks and creates images."

Visualization is a natural gift everyone possesses and can utilize. Unfortunately, television, video and cinema have undermined the free creative play of our spirit. We are fed finished images that leave no space for imagination; hence our powers of imagination have dwindled. However, our potential for creative imagining can be activated by reading suitable literature and by practicing the following exercise.

Visualization exercise

We think in images more than in words. Choose a simple object such as a stone or a flower, and imprint its image in your mind. Then, set aside the chosen object, close your eyes, and allow it to reappear in your mind. The first step in chakra breathing is to focus on the chakra you are working with. The more you exercise your perceptive and imaginative capacities, the easier you will find working with your chakras.

Use the same process to open the chakras. Imagine each chakra opening. By doing this, your imagination will initiate the process of activating and balancing the centers.

Then, direct your breath into the chakra. Imagine the diameter of the chakra expanding. Visualize the chakras pulsating, circling, and flowing with increased power, and imagine the basic colors of each chakra shining more brilliantly than before.

Exercise postures

With one exception (see illustrations) the traditional postures for chakra breathing are either kneeling or cross-legged.

However, if you have back or leg problems, a straight-back chair is equally acceptable. Lay the backs of your hands on your thighs, keeping your hands relaxed. If you use a chair, make sure the soles of your feet are firmly planted on the floor.

If, for whatever reason, you can only relax fully while lying on your back, then make this position as comfortable as possible for yourself. This applies only to the first chakra breathing exercise.

Close your eyes before beginning, and keep them closed throughout. Closing your eyes will help you gain insight into your inner world—a world of feelings and sensations. Like nomads, our eyes are constantly wandering.

Practice schedule for the first three weeks

If this is your first experience of breathing practice, I would suggest you use the following schedule:

Days one through three:

Practice inner mindfulness while watching the breath. Watch your breath several times a day for about ten minutes at a time. Watching does not mean interfering with the process. Rather, watching means accepting whatever happens without judgment.

Days four through seven:

Active breathing and visualizing

Lying on your back, take 30 slow, deep inhalations and exhalations several times a day. Pay close attention to the exhalations. Also, use the previously described exercise to train your imagination and ability to visualize.

Days eight through fourteen:

Begin practicing the first chakra exercise.

Practice it for a week, or until you feel confident and secure with the increased level of energy. Practice only once a day. Try to stay conscious of every slight change within your body and mind. Gradually familiarize yourself with the second chakra exercise.

Days fifteen through twenty-one:

Practice both chakra exercises daily. After twenty-one days, practicing the breathing exercises two or three times a week is generally sufficient.

Advanced practice schedule

Practice makes perfect! Ideally, you should practice in the morning after waking up, and again in the late afternoon, two or three times a week. Do not practice immediately before going to bed. The activated energy stimulates the nervous system and may prevent you from falling asleep.

I will now introduce the two chakra breathing exercises and help familiarize you with them. The morning exercise activates the energy centers, while the afternoon exercise balances them.

Chapter 7

Practice With
Patience and Self-Respect

Benefits of chakra breathing practice:

Enlivening of all energy centers and physical energies, heightening of energetic vibrations to their optimal frequency, dissolution of tensions and energy blockages, calming and clearing of the mind, physical and mental purification, increased inner stillness and serenity in daily life, more alertness and consciousness of sensations in the present moment, awareness of one's center, harmonizing of the entire nervous system and the most important secretory glands.

Breathing meditation

This short breathing meditation will familiarize you with your breathing and your energy. Sit straight and relax. Close your eyes and observe your breathing. Let your breath come and go easily and naturally for the duration of about ten breaths. Then inhale and exhale thirty times deeply and evenly, maintaining full awareness.

Quiet meditation and relaxation

To complete both chakra breathing exercises, remain seated for a few minutes after the phase of active breathing.

Close your eyes as you exhale. Sit straight and listen into yourself. Watch your breathing carefully.

At this stage, you should remain completely passive. Do nothing. Simply allow the presence of whatever arises on its own. Enjoy the experience of doing nothing and wanting nothing.

Then lie down on your back, and give the weight of your body to the earth. Feel yourself being carried, safe and protected. Breath quietly and easily. Let go—let yourself drop. Feel one with yourself, with nature and the earth.

Chapter 8

Breathing Exercise 1
Afternoon Meditation

This exercise is used in the late afternoon to harmonize the subtle energy centers. It has a gentler and more relaxing effect than Breathing Exercise 2, which is used in the morning.

Breath gently, choosing a speed which allows you to be conscious in every moment. Please do not hurry and avoid pumping your lungs full of air forcefully.

Slow inhalations increase our ability to perceive details clearly. Avoid forcing out the breath on the exhalation. Leave the process of exhaling to your body. Inhalation and exhalation need to come into harmonious relationship. Thus the two poles of exhaling and inhaling become one—a single sound or note, uniting yin and yang. This causes profound feelings of release and relaxation.

Breathe slowly, evenly, staying relaxed. Throughout the exercise, honor your personal limitations. If you should feel dizzy or confused, reduce the depth of your breathing.

Follow these five steps:

1. First, do the breathing meditation. (p. 65-66) which will familiarize you with your breathing process and guide you to a deeper level of relaxation. Remember, the preliminary meditation consists of observing your breath quietly for a while, taking about ten to fifteen breaths. Then, breathe deeply and evenly for about thirty breaths without pausing. Allow the exhalations to happen naturally, letting your body take over

Now take a few minutes to listen into yourself. Do not try to channel your energy during these moments of relaxation, but simply experience the inner streaming. Do not "do" anything actively now, but simply enjoy your being.

2. Now, begin by bringing your attention toward and into the first chakra. Use your imagination to visualize the chakra opening.

3. Breathe in a four-count rhythm, taking three shorter breaths and one longer one. Chakra breathing is a gentle, harmonious process. There are no gaps between breaths. In your imagination, allow the chakra to unfold, and breathe into it for three to five minutes.

4. Rest for about a minute, letting the chakra unfold. (If you are practicing with a chakra breathing tape, simply follow the instructions.) Then move on to the next chakra.

5. After breathing into the last chakra—the crown chakra—move into the closing quiet meditation and relaxation, as described on page 66. After sitting peacefully, lie down comfortably on your back and visualize a warm, healing light in and around each chakra. Allow your energy to flow freely, without directing or controlling anything.

Chapter 9

Breathing Exercise 2
Morning Meditation

This exercise is used in the morning to activate and harmonize the subtle energy centers. Use the following procedure for all seven chakras. Like the first, it begins with the preliminary breathing meditation.

For each chakra, assume the breathing posture indicated by the illustration. Take about thirty seconds to focus your attention on the center you are about to breath into.

Then breathe in and out through your nose quickly and forcefully for about sixty seconds. There are a few exceptions—refer to the illustrations. After this stage of active breathing, inhale deeply one more time, then hold the breath as long as you can.

Relax as you exhale and listen within. The moments immediately after the active phase of breathing are extremely conducive to increased self-awareness, perception and insight . Only by keeping your mind on the here and now can you perceive your inner process and be aware of the quality of your breathing.

Close the chakra mentally. The movements for each position are given with the illustrations.

Rest for about one minute before moving on to activate the next chakra.

Conclude with the quiet meditation and relax-ation previously described.

Opening breathing meditation

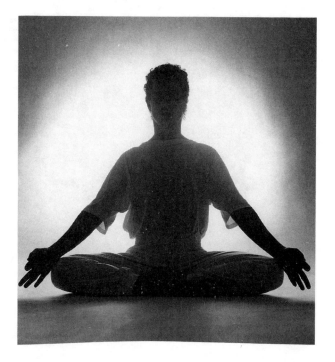

Sit straight and relax. Close your eyes and observe your breathing. Let your breath come and go easily and naturally for the duration of about ten breaths. Then inhale and exhale deeply and evenly, thirty times, maintaining full awareness.

Root chakra

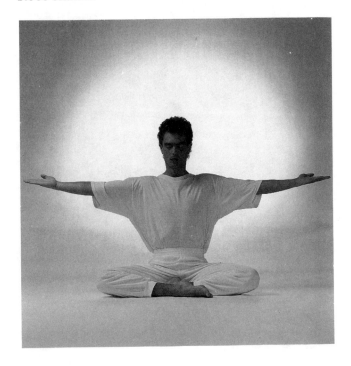

Kneel or sit cross-legged. Stretch your arms out to the side, holding them at the height of your shoulders. Your palms should face upward. With every inhalation and exhalation, your hands move up and down like little wings.

Navel chakra

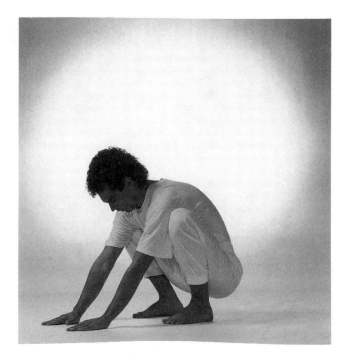

Squat, keeping the soles of your feet in full contact with the ground, so that you are sitting between your legs. Stretch your arms forward, and place your palms on the ground. If you find it difficult to maintain balance, lean against a wall. Allow your head to relax and drop down.

Solar plexus

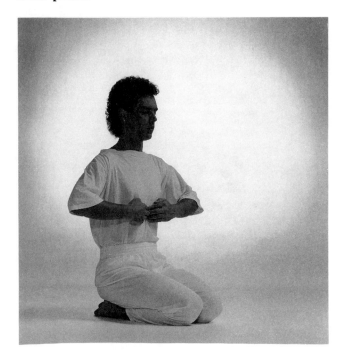

Kneel. Place the fingertips of both hands on your solar plexus. On every exhalation, allow your upper torso to bend forward slightly, like a hinge. Straighten your body as you inhale.

Heart chakra

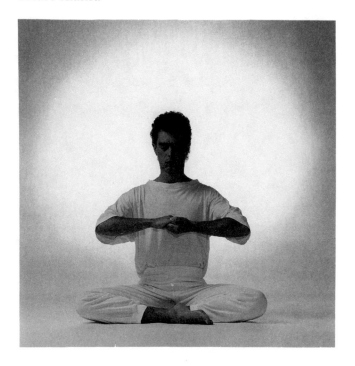

Kneel or sit cross-legged. Hook the fingers of your hands together at the level of your heart and gently pull outwards. Your hands and arms form a straight line. Your elbows rise and fall, swinging up and down with the rhythm of your breath.

Throat chakra

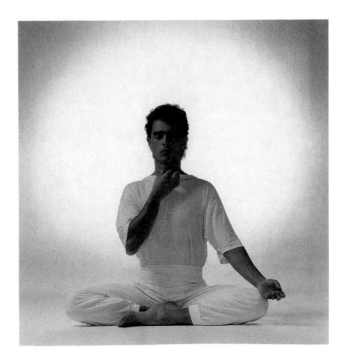

Kneel or sit cross-legged. Feel the location of your throat; then lay your hands on your thighs. Inhale quickly and forcefully twice through your nose, then exhale twice in the same manner through your mouth, imitating a locomotive.

Third eye chakra

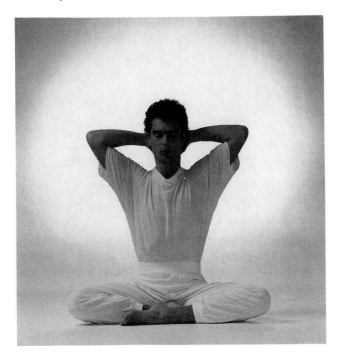

Kneel or sit cross-legged. Cross your hands behind
your head. On the inhalation, pull your elbows
back, on the exhalation, move them to the front.

Crown chakra

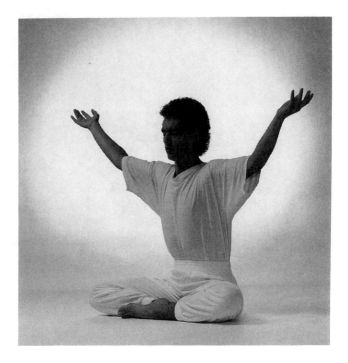

Kneel or sit cross-legged. Stretch your arms up
above your head. Breathe in and out through your
nose with a sniffing sound. Stay mindful. After a
short pause, visualize a healing, warm, radiant light
in and around each chakra.

Meditation and rest phase

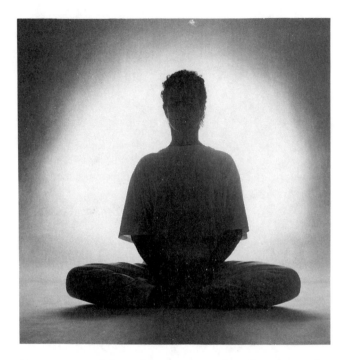

Remain seated for a few minutes after the phase of active breathing. Close your eyes as you exhale. Sit straight and listen into yourself. Watch your breathing carefully, remaining completely passive. Allow the presence of whatever arises on its own. Enjoy the openness of doing nothing and wanting nothing.

Sitting quietly, doing nothing, spring comes and the grass grows by itself.

Zen saying

Relaxation phase

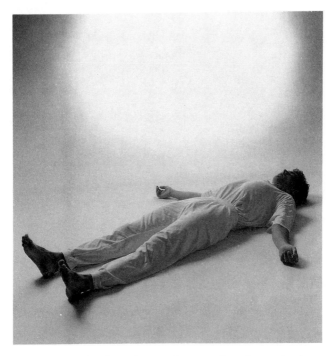

Lie on your back and give the weight of your body
to the earth. Feel yourself being carried, safe and
protected. Breath quietly and easily. Let go—let
yourself drop. Feel one with yourself, with nature
and the earth.

Epilogue

The adventure of breathing

The journey into oneself is a leap into the unknown. When we try to discover our potential and to find out who we truly are, we embark on an adventurous path, feeling our way through the darkness toward the light —a true quest.

The inner world offers a great deal of information concerning what is really going on within. In the course of time your awareness of breath and body, your sensitivity and insight into your true feelings and sensations will undoubtedly increase.

Your breath is the bridge to new insights and to a sense of well-being. Breathing opens a window into another world. Again and again, we experience conscious breathing bestowing a sense of safety upon us, dissolving limitations and leading us into other dimensions of existence. Breath can carry us back to the source, the source we call life and being.

On this path, I myself rediscovered my faith in life—a trust that everything happens in accordance with a deep inner plan.

We live in this world in order to become increasingly whole and light. Whenever we reach a boundary at which laziness or fear could hold us back from further progress in our personal evolution, breath serves as a valuable ally and as a powerful catalyst for change.

Honoring and befriending your breath

These exercises will help you to become a more conscious and mindful participant in life's process. Trust your breath. It is one of the most powerful sources of life you possess. Though we take our breathing for granted, it is absolutely essential to life. Unfortunately, we tend to undervalue whatever we have in abundant quantities, especially if it is invisible like oxygen. Though we breathe unconsciously, taking our breath for granted, each breath is nonetheless a gift.

The chakra breathing exercises are so simple that anyone can practice them, yet they have the power to gently revitalize and harmonize all the energy centers. As you know, this can only occur with the help of regular practice.

We know from experience that to achieve or change something in our life, we must initially be willing to dedicate more time and attention to reaching this goal than we do to our more routine activities. We need to practice. Consider whether you are willing to nurture yourself in this way, fostering your sensitivity and patience.

After some time, you will find yourself able to heal your physical and subtle levels of energy and to create a harmonious state of balance among the energies within you.

Open to your feelings. If you want to get acquainted with your own inner life, you should take time to listen to yourself, accept and encounter yourself. A rich world of sensations and emotions will reveal itself.

Invite breath to become your best friend—it already is, though you may not yet be aware of it. Your breath will support and transform you in miraculous ways, and will teach you to accept both yourself and the natural cycles of life. It will lead you on an extremely interesting journey and help you realize the human being you really are—a divine being.

My best wishes go with you.

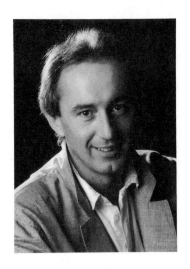

About the Author

Helmut G. Sieczka is a breathing teacher, a certified rebirther, and author of several books. He has worked in the field of humanistic therapy for over ten years, and leads workshops throughout Europe which focus on spiritual evolution and the expansion of consciousness.

Order Form

CHAKRA BREATHING CASSETTE

Guided exercises for daily breathing meditation
opening, balancing, and unfolding the chakras.

Chakra Breathing Cassette	$12.95
Mailing	1.50
California residents only add 7.25% sales tax	.94
Total Enclosed	

Name

Address

City   State   Zip

Make check payable to LifeRhythm, or use your credit card.
International orders add $3 for surface mail and $5 for
airmail; pay by International Money Order or by check
drawn on a U.S. Bank.

LifeRhythm

P.O. Box 806   Mendocino CA 95460   USA
Tel: (707) 937-1825 Fax: (707) 937-3052
http://www.liferhythm.com   books@liferhythm.com

LIFERHYTHM PUBLICATIONS

John C. Pierrakos, M.D. CORE ENERGETICS
Developing the Capacity to Love and Heal
With 16 pages of four-color illustrations of human auras corresponding to their character structure, 300 pages, $18.95
Honored psychiatrist, body-therapist, and authority on consciousness and human energy fields, John C. Pierrakos, M.D. founded the Core Energetic therapeutic movement. In this classic text, Dr. Pierrakos discusses opening the "Core" to heal people and bring them to a new awareness and unification of body, emotions, mind, will, and spirit.

John C. Pierrakos M.D. EROS, LOVE & SEXUALITY
The Unifying Forces of Life and Relationship
150 pages
In this long awaited book, John C. Pierrakos, M.D. discusses three different aspects of the one life force that generates all activity and creativity. When we are open, we experience the forces of eros, love and sexuality as one. A student and collegue of Wilhelm Reich, Dr. Pierrakos co-founded Bioenergetics and later developed Core Energetics.

Malcolm Brown, Ph.D. THE HEALING TOUCH
An Introduction to Organismic Psychotherapy
320 pages 38 illustrations
A moving and meticulous account of Malcolm Brown's journey from Rogerian-style verbal psychotherapist to gifted body psychotherapist. Dr. Brown developed his own art and science of body psychotherapy with the purpose of re-activating the natural mental/spiritual polarities of the embodied soul and transcendental psyche. Using powerful case histories as examples, Brown describes the theory, practice and development of his work.

Bodo Baginski & Shalila Sharamon   REIKI   Universal Life Energy
200 pages   illustrations
With the help of specific methods, anyone can learn to awaken and
activate this universal life energy so that healing and harmonizing
energy flows through the hands. This book features a unique com-
pilation and interpretation from the author's experience of over 200
psychosomatic symptoms and diseases

Fran Brown   LIVING REIKI: TAKATA'S TEACHINGS
Stories from the Life of Hawayo Takata
110 pages
In this loving memoir to her teacher, Fran Brown gathered the col-
orful stories told by Hawayo Takata during her thirty-five years as
the only teaching Reiki Master. Fran Brown's accounts create an
inspirational panorama of Takata's teachings, filled with practical
and spiritual aspects of a life given to healing.

Bridgitte Müller & Horst Günther
A COMPLETE BOOK OF REIKI HEALING
Heal Yourself, Others, and the World Around You
192 pages, 85 photographs and illustrations
Europe's first Reiki Master, Brigitte Müller writes about her opening
into a new world of healing with the freshness of discovery. Horst
Günther's experience of Reiki at one of Brigitte's first workshops in
Germany changed the course of his life. Together they share a vision
of universal life energy and the use of Reiki to help us heal ourselves
and each other. Complete with Reiki history and practice, photographs, drawings, and clear hand placement instructions.

Ron Kurtz   BODY-CENTERED   PSYCHOTHERAPY:
THE HAKOMI METHOD
The Integrated Use of Mindfulness, Nonviolence and the Body
212 pages, illustrations
Hakomi bodywork stems from a synthesis of philospohies: Bud-
dhism, Taoism, and the general systems theory, which incorporates
respect for the wisdom of each individual as a living organic system
organizing the needed matter and energy to sustain itself.

R. Stamboliev   THE ENERGETICS OF VOICE
                  DIALOGUE

Exploring the Energetics of Transformational Psychology
100 pages

The work of PhDs Hal and Sidra Stone, Voice Dialogue bases therapy on the transformational model of consciousness, approaching
the human psyche as a synthesis of experience-patterns that can be
changed. Transformation can only occur when the original pattern
of an experience is touched, understood and felt from the adult, integrated perspective of an "Aware Ego." Offering exercises to develop therapeutic skills, this book explores the energetic relationship
between client and therapist, and illustrates with case histories.

Cousto   THE COSMIC OCTAVE
           Origin of Harmony

128 pages, 45 illustrations, numerous tables, 24 page appendix
Cousto demonstrates the direct relationship of astronomical data,
such as the frequency of planetary orbits to ancient and modern
measuring systems, the human body, music and medicine. *Please
ask for special information about Cosmic Octave Tuning Forks,
available only from LifeRhythm.* These high quality German-made
healing tools are calibrated to the planets: Mercury, Venus, Mars,
Jupiter, Saturn, Uranus, Neptune, Pluto, the Sun, Sidereal Earth,
Platonic Earth, Earth Year (OM), Synoptic Moon, and Sidereral
Moon.

R. Flatischler   THE FORGOTTEN POWER OF RHYTHM
TA KE TI NA

160 pages, illustrations, supplemental CD or cassette available
Rhythm—the central power of our lives—connects us all. Reinhard
Flatischler presents his brilliant approach to rhythm is this book, for
both the lay-person and the professional musician, providing a new
understanding of the many musical voices on the planet. The TA
KE TI NA expereince offers the interaction of pulse, breath, voice,
walking and clapping, awakening our inherent rhythm in the most
direct way—through the body.

LifeRhythm

Connects you with your Core and entire being—guided by Science, Intuition and Love.

We provide tools for growth, therapy, holistic health and higher education through publications, seminars and workshops.

If you are interested in our forthcoming projects and want to be on our mailing list, send your address to:

LifeRhythm
PO Box 806 Mendocino CA 95460
Tel: (707) 937-1825 Fax: (707) 937-3052
email: books@liferhythm.com
http://www.liferhythm.com